Contents

Prologue 2

Sitting MRCP Part 2 and PACES simultaneously 5

Before We Start 7

Joining a PACES Group 9

Consultant and Registrar Teaching Rota 11

Knowledge, Practice and Presentation 13

Marginal Gains, Deliberate Practice & Accumulation 15

Proposed PACES 2021 format 20

❋ PACES Triangle 22

Invest in a great course 34

Weeks 1 and 2 37

Week 3 41

Creating systematic presentations 45

Weeks 4, 5 and 6 49

Weeks 7 and 8 54

MRCP PACES Marking Scheme 56

Read the scenario. Then read it again. 60

Non-technical skills 62

PACES Fast Track & Failing 63

Prologue

MRCP PACES is usually the final hurdle between you and the much coveted MRCP diploma.

At this career stage you probably feel that your social and work lives are blurring and have been consumed by MRCP. You may also feel that the only thing between you and a consultant post is these nine letters.

If that sounds like you then I can hardly blame you. I remember being in this situation in 2015 right before I sat PACES in Edinburgh but to be honest, life continues regardless the outcome of your exam. A useful tip to curb anxiety before a major life-event such as MRCP PACES or the delivering of an important presentation is to imagine your surroundings ten, twenty or even one hundred years from now when everyone including yourself will no longer be on the planet. The building you're currently in might still be here, occupied by different people but the events that happen today are very relatively insignificant in the grand scheme of things. Practicing this type of thought experiment can be very humbling.

By the end of CT2, some of us can perform internal jugular vein cannulations and intercostal chest drains (ICDs) with relative ease but you'll soon realise that being a specialty registrar is a lot more than this.

During my time as a respiratory CT2, I remember having placed what must've been about twenty 12Fr chest drains into large malignant pleural effusions. In hindsight, my consultants must've selected these patients for me based on perceived and thereafter actual ease of procedure. I thought every ICD was straightforward. However, once I started ST3, I realised that medicine is a far more nuanced art and science than first meets the eye. Like most endeavours, the more you know about a subject, the more you realise you don't know. Almost like you've reached a level of competence where you're aware of your areas of incompetence.

Nowadays I anticipate placing difficult 26Fr ICDs into complicated empyemas and competently managing complex outpatient respiratory patients. I have also recently entered a clinical research post and am pursuing a higher MD degree in airways disease.

The purpose of telling you about my career progression is that hopefully it will place your circumstance into perspective. At one point you were maybe preoccupied with high school exams, and your prospects for entering medical school were uncertain. Or perhaps upon passing your medical school finals and you worried yourself with foundation jobs. MRCP PACES is simply another career checkpoint every physician must overcome at one point in their lives. **You may fail, but you'll probably pass if you diligently implement everything in this guide, but in the end it does not really matter.**

By seeing MRCP PACES as only a checkpoint in your very long journey in becoming the best physician you can be, hopefully you'll understand that it's not the Mount Everest everyone makes it out to be. Almost everyone eventually passes and goes on to become a consultant in their field.

This guide will walk you through what you need to do to maximise your chances of **passing PACES on your first attempt and in just 8 weeks**.

Sitting MRCP Part 2 and PACES simultaneously

*"Think back to a time when nursing staff approached you one after another with prescription charts, observation charts and fluid charts. Literally queuing up like customers at a lemonade stand. Your FY1 then runs into the room asking you about a gentleman who is vomiting bowlfuls of frank red blood. That's what attempting MRCP PACES and Part 2 **simultaneously** feels like."*

I overheard a consultant say that to one of the core medical trainees (CMTs) once.

As individuals we're all capable of extreme feats, but we almost never use the full extent of our potential. For example, of those who are not regular runners, how many of you believe you could complete a marathon next week with little to no training? The vast majority of us would actually be able to – we might not necessarily achieve a very respectable finish time, but we would finish nevertheless, if some weight was attached to it. We would run, walk or even crawl over that finish line if something depended on it. For most of our lives we are running on about 40% of our potential so imagine what we can achieve if we decided to just hang in there.

I personally chose not to sit MRCP Part 2 and PACES simultaneously. One of my fellow CMTs managed this feat in 2015 whilst tackling the practical driving test because she would not have been able to take up a ST3 post otherwise. If you find yourself in this situation i.e. late CT2 or what would now be considered IMY3 soon, then you need to believe in yourself.

I still believe the ideal situation is to sit these exams consecutively and not simultaneously as they test different facets of your knowledge and have completely different formats. Although it would be extremely pleasant to attain complete MRCP diploma in FY2 for example, this does not realistically confer you a head-start in terms of career progression. You'll still need to undergo IMY1 – 3 prior to ST3/4 initiation. You should always strive to enjoy the process and journey at least a little and try to not to ruminate about the destination.

PACES tests your real-time ability to perform under pressure as well as your communication skills and interaction with patients and relatives.

The majority of you reading this guide will have already passed Part 2 and I congratulate you for having come so far. For those who are contemplating both exams together, it's certainly possible to pass both exams simultaneously, especially if you have the correct motivation in place. However, if you can afford the option, take a slightly slower pace as it ultimately does not grant you a faster career progression in most cases.

Before We Start

"Work expands so as to fill the time available for its completion."

Parkinson's Law is the reason why 8 weeks is enough time for PACES. Most of us are familiar with being given a few weeks for a piece of university coursework, only to complete it at lightning speed in the last couple of days before due date. Parkinson's law particularly resonated with me during third year of medical school when we were assigned a piece of coursework with a deadline of two months. I ended up doing an all-nighter inside the university library the night before, cramming in 60 days of work in 10 hours!

After completing MRCP Parts 1 and 2 Written I decided to leave 7 months until my PACES attempt in July 2015. Instead of starting my revision immediately, I celebrated completion of the two exams with a holiday to Japan with my then girlfriend. Upon return and presumably still in holiday mode I completely lost motivation and interest and began cruising auto-pilot through the remainder of my first core medical training year. I did not participate in the **concept of deliberate practice** and went to work every day without showing enthusiasm to learn or do anything new. Surprisingly and unfortunately a lot of the trainees I work with nowadays give off this impression.

It wasn't until end of April I decided to properly start my preparation. It was during this 8-week period I took control of the steering wheel and ended up passing in early July 2015 on my first attempt.

This guide documents the eight week period in my life when I took advantage of our friend Parkinson. This is the 8-week technique you can use to clear PACES so you can concentrate on more important things in life, like spending time with your kids, or learning a new registrar skill like endoscopy. But remember to try and enjoy the process because although you will pass PACES, there will undoubtedly be another PACES-like endeavour in your life. Learn to enjoy the struggle however ridiculous it may sound.

Before we start, we are going to carry out **two tasks**. The first is to find a **motivated study group or a partner** and the **second is to invest in a great course**.

Joining a PACES Group

"You're the average of the five people you spend most time with."

This is one of my favourite quotes of all time because it's simple yet so true. Success breeds success and a culture of failure breeds nothing but more failure and toxicity.

How can you fully harness the power of that quote?

The first piece of homework you have is advertising to your colleagues, registrars and consultants that you're attempting PACES in x months. In addition to placing some pressure and accountability onto yourself, people are generally very helpful and will suggest going to a specific registrar or consultant who is very keen to teach. Alternatively, they will know at least someone who is currently on the same path as you. One of the most useful items is something akin to a PACES whatsapp group where you can exchange ideas and arrange revision sessions.

The best study partner is someone who is somewhat more motivated than you but not over-anxious about the exam. The accountability of having to turn up to a revision session is always useful. Remember you want that sweet spot where there is a certain amount of urgency, but not too much.

The other piece of advice is to switch any music you listen to for medical audio, in the form of podcasts or videos when you are doing activities that don't require much thought i.e. listening to podcasts on your daily commute to work or watching a video on the ophthalmology examination whilst on the treadmill. This is indeed an inadvertent way of surrounding yourself with like-minded people using technology and is a massive advantage that only technology has made possible.

Consultant and Registrar Teaching Rota

If you work at a small hospital and can't find anyone to study with, now is the time to be proactive. You have the option to listen to **PACES podcasts** which are freely available, in essence surrounding yourself with like-minded people. It's always useful to learn about how others think through problems and presentations. Ask your local or regional education department who might be able to point you in the right direction.

You also have the option to create your own PACES study group, with you as the first member. If you work in a small hospital you may have to invite or join a group from another hospital from the same trust. If your desire to pass MRCP is strong enough, traveling twice a week after work to another hospital is something you'll have to do. It can't be stressed enough how important **group study** is for PACES. Although there is some strategy to Parts 1 and 2 at least you can still force a pass with enough effort. For PACES you'll struggle with just book study as you need to continuously critique each other's demeanour and communication skills throughout these 8 weeks to simulate exam conditions.

Something else to consider is a **consultant and registrar teaching rota**. Again, if this isn't available locally, be proactive and create one, or join one from another hospital in your trust.

Ideally you want to create a "double sided rota" where you have experienced consultants and senior registrars imparting their specialist wisdom. You'll understand when I say that some things simply cannot be learned from books and this is where their experience and discussions become critical. The second side to your rota should contain CT2s and junior registrars who have recently completed their PACES exam and can therefore teach you invaluable tips and tricks. Imagine having someone who has just sat the exam at the same venue you'll be sitting PACES in.

Knowledge, Practice and Presentation

Now onto information that will increase your chances of overcoming PACES.

PACES is difficult not because of the depth of knowledge required. In fact, due to **time restraints** and **choice of examiner**, you can only ever be asked what a general physician should be expected to know about a given subject.

PACES is proposed to be reformatted in 2021 due to COVID (originally 2020) to more reflect real life clinical practice and overall this is a good thing. There will be two 20-minute stations (stations 2 and 5) that assess all seven skills essentially giving candidates 15 minutes for history and examination, and 5 minutes for examiner questions and your answers. If you play your cards strategically your examiner should really only have time to ask 3 or 4 questions. Likewise, in the new examination stations (stations 1, 3 and 4) 4 minutes for questions should equate to a maximum of 3 examiner questions.

Secondly, choice of examiner refers to the fact that the exam board would never ask a respiratory physician to examine you at the respiratory station nor would you find a gastroenterologist grilling you about hepatitis. It's recognised that this would obviously be unfair to candidates as examiners would inadvertently or subconsciously ask far more difficult questions that a generalist would not necessarily be expected to know. You'll most likely have two generalists at each station i.e.

a cardiologist examining you at the renal station and an elderly physician examining you in the respiratory station.

Knowing the above, you should start your revision using what I call the **PACES Triangle**: knowledge, practice and presentation.

Marginal Gains, Deliberate Practice & Accumulation

When we watch great snooker players such as Stephen Hendry or super chess grandmasters like Magnus Carlsen, they make their game look so effortless. In a tournament they can wipe the floor with their opponents; their actions so natural most people regard them as talented to the extent of unachievable.

Of course, these exceptional people are ultra-talented and not anyone off the street could play to that level irrespective the number of hours they put in. What we don't see, however, are the hours upon hours of practice they endure (or enjoy) behind the scenes before the curtain is finally lifted and the lights are shining.

Closer examination of their practice routines will reveal that the concept of **deliberate practice** is at play. For instance, you would not find Hendry mindlessly poking snooker balls in his prime, nor Carlsen half-heartedly making chess moves. This is unfortunately what most of us do when we "practice" a specific sport. For most of us practising basketball would mainly involve throwing the ball into the hoop repeatedly as that generates instant gratification and feedback. A more serious basketball player might recognise the importance of cardiovascular fitness and as a result spend more time on the treadmill. A basketball star would breakdown and optimise every facet of the game down to dribbling, footwork and nutrition, recognising that without these he may not even get the opportunity to shoot the winning shot.

Deliberate practice is intense, not instantly gratifying and some aspects of it can be very onerous. Even though you might love the game of basketball, nobody wants to spend every minute off the court dialling in perfect recovery in the form of sleep and nutrition. But this is what you have to do to succeed.

PACES is not simply an examination of your clinical knowledge, otherwise pass rates would be a lot higher. 95% of us have the necessary knowledge but like in a practical driving exam, you have to be able to demonstrate this and also justify your actions to the examiners. To improve your chances of passing PACES you will have to breakdown and optimise every facet of the exam just like the basketball professional breaks down their game. There is little point in performing the half-hearted respiratory examination we all do during the ward round – let's face it, when was the last time percussion changed your investigation or management plan? Instead you will need to painstakingly look at every finger for clubbing, gentle palpate every trachea for deviation and percuss every chest for dullness. You will need to breakdown the exam in terms of your own body language and tonality, timing and mindset. Deliberate practice is very difficult, and you may find that the number of hours you're able to implement this will drastically reduce. However, it is far more effective and much more likely to pay dividends for you.

If we return to the giants of chess, snooker and basketball, many people often assume that success is one huge event, like winning the world championship or scoring that victorious point in the last minute of a match. But in reality, to reach that level, you must rely on **marginal gains** – there is no other option.

Marginal gains refers to small incremental checkpoints you achieve day in day out. For example, choosing a cup of water instead of a can of soda would be a simple marginal gain.

Although it sounds simple to implement (anyone can drink a cup of water) marginal gains will not change the person you are overnight or even after a week. Choosing that healthy meal over fast food will not make you healthy overnight which is why the obesity epidemic and other comorbidities such as hypertension and diabetes are so prevalent. Even after one month of eating clean you might not notice much difference in front of the mirror although of course this depends on your starting point.

However, as the months roll by, you will certainly notice a big difference after 1 year, which ultimately isn't that much time. Brewing your own coffee won't make you rich overnight but that £2 saved daily becomes £700 in one year.

Depending on how you look at it, one of the tragedies or wonders of this world is the concept of **accumulation**. If you choose to drink water instead of soda every day, you might find it easier to stay at a healthy weight. This undoubtedly makes you more attractive and finding a partner will be more effortless. If you choose to drink soda every day your weight will most likely skyrocket, making it more difficult to find a desirable partner. This in turn might lead to a downward spiral in terms of mental health and subsequent binge eating, further worsening your weight and health.

If you choose to brew your coffee, that £2 saved is not just £700 in cash a year, but £700 of opportunity a year. That £700 can act as an emergency fund in case of unexpected events or it can be applied to investing where a realistic 7% return will give you an extra £49 a year.

Essentially the rich (in any sense) get richer and well, the poor unfortunately get poorer.

If we apply **marginal gains** to PACES, every aspect of your preparation will ultimately determine your result. You must divide your preparation into basic blocks with the knowledge aspect only being one block – remember that's a given – that 95% of you will know the material by the time of the exam. Why is the fail rate so high? People who fail normally neglect other aspects of preparation like having proper structure, keeping strictly to timing, presentation skills, body language, diet and sleep etc. If you apply marginal gains and improve every aspect of your PACES ability by 1% every day, you'll have improved by 74.5% after 8 weeks. *

Adhering to **deliberate practice** goes hand in hand with marginal gains. There is little point in turning up to study sessions if you're half asleep. Just putting in the hours is not enough as the quality of those hours is what's important. I personally prefer not studying rather than working for 10 minutes, spending 20 minutes on youtube and then studying for another 5 minutes before booting up the Xbox. At least when you're not studying you stay true to yourself. Everything you do towards PACES should be deliberate and you should be able to justify why you're doing it.

Finally, although the daily effects of your actions might not appear profound, the cumulative effects will shock you at the end of your 8 weeks. As you become more competent you may find yourself shifting from the paradigm of unconscious incompetence to conscious competence and ultimately to unconscious competence.

* Calculated by 1.01^56

Proposed PACES 2021 format

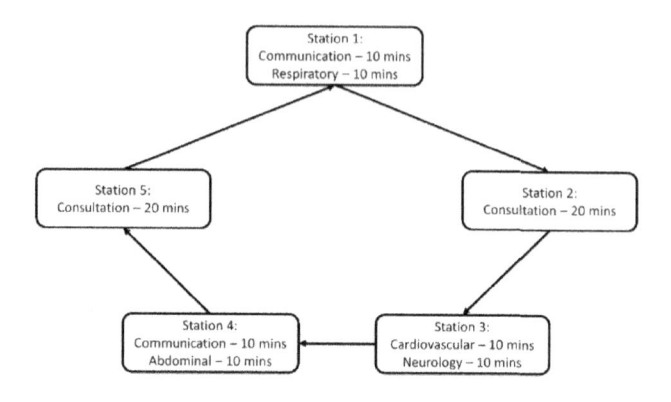

Figure 1 Proposed PACES 2021 format

From 2021 onwards, figure 1 best demonstrates the new PACES carousel. Each box represents a 20-minute station and therefore each carousel usually consists of five candidates. You may find yourself starting at station 2 for example, but the directional arrows indicate that your journey will be through stations 3, 4, 5 and finally 1. Each station is separated by a 5-minute "break" which factors in time for you to read the scenario for your next station. The entire exam usually takes 125 minutes.

Compared to the current PACES format (figure 2) we notice that the history taking station 2 may be removed due to a feeling that isolated history taking is artificial in modern clinical practice. The communications skills and ethics station 4 may also been removed as it is felt to be rather excessive and offers less value than the other stations in terms of overall assessment. Although station 5 is arguably the most "real-life" aspect of PACES, ten minutes per scenario feel very rushed and pressurised.

[In new stations 1 and 4, a 10-minute communication encounter may be introduced, with the main highlight being that there will be no question and answer section from the examiners. This section will be judged on observation alone. Depending on the way you view the new format, station 5 will in the future be divided into two separate 20-minute consultation encounters (stations 2 and 5) where all seven skills are assessed. There will be 15 minutes for structured history, physical examination, explanation of diagnosis and management, and addressing questions or concerns. This will be followed by a 5-minute question and answer section with the examiners.]

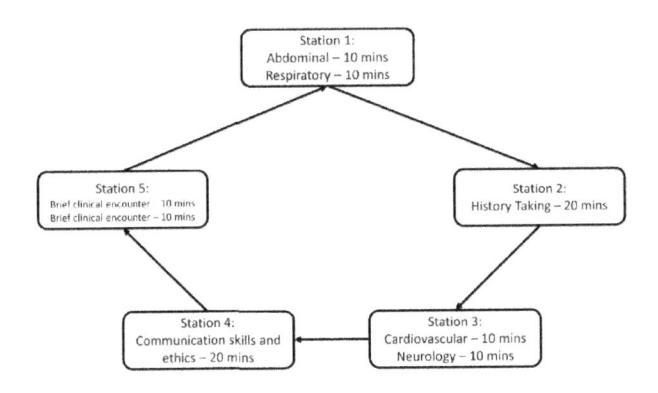

```
                    Station 1:
                Abdominal – 10 mins
                Respiratory – 10 mins

   Station 5:                         Station 2:
Brief clinical encounter 10 mins    History Taking – 20 mins
Brief clinical encounter – 10 mins

        Station 4:                  Station 3:
   Communication skills and     Cardiovascular – 10 mins
       ethics – 20 mins           Neurology – 10 mins
```

Figure 2 Current PACES format

Figure 2 depicts the <u>current</u> PACES format that all candidates should be familiar with.

PACES Triangle

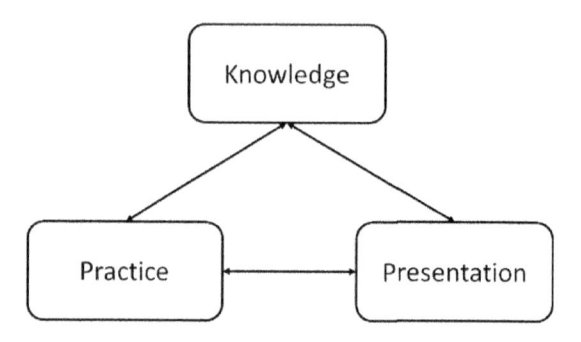

Figure 3 The PACES Triangle

As with MRCP Parts 1 and 2 written, accruing knowledge should be your initial goal. Without it you're unable to demonstrate your ability to the examiners regardless of how charismatic or practised you are. Knowledge is the foundation and cement with which you will build your castle. As you study for PACES you'll find that a significant amount of knowledge you gained from the written exams will hold you in good stead in front of the examiners during question time. This so-called **theoretical knowledge** is especially useful when it comes to pattern recognition, making diagnoses and management plans and answering examiner questions. However, theoretical knowledge can only take you so far in a directly observed examination of clinical skills which is why the pass rate for PACES remains low. In addition to knowledge of theory, you'll therefore also need to accrue **practical knowledge**.

The books I would recommend for PACES-specific practical knowledge are both the volumes of Clinical Medicine for the MRCP PACES by Mehta, Iqbal and Bowman. They contain comprehensive descriptions of common signs for most of the conditions you'll likely encounter in PACES and have strong clinically based answers for the likely questions that you might be asked. I would highly recommend using this book for the physical examination stations (1 and 3) for nothing else but to learn the catchphrases and ten-pound words used to present signs to the examiners.

Although now touching upon the presentation apex of the PACES triangle, the concept of **taking initiative** in this exam cannot be stressed enough. Consider the following exchange between examiner and candidate:

E: You mentioned the differential diagnosis includes pulmonary fibrosis and bronchiectasis. Why is that?

C: Yes, due to the presence of bilateral crepitations in both bases.

E: So how would you differentiate between them?

C: I would request a chest x-ray, spirometry and perhaps a CT chest.

E: And what would you expect to find?

When sitting any exam, knowledge is undoubtedly of paramount importance representing the peak of the PACES triangle. In the above exchange, sure the candidate can answer all the examiner's questions and their knowledge base is adequate. However, if you place yourself in the shoes of the examiner, the above exchange is very tedious even if this was the first candidate of the day. As one of the organising registrars for multiple PACES exams in Scotland, I realised that most examiners are looking to pass candidates, but candidates must help themselves first and foremost. Remember to aim for the path of least resistance even if it means more effort on your part.

Instead of making question and answer time a soul-destroying exercise for everyone in the party, we can perhaps make an adjustment:

C: *After presentation of patient case* Therefore I feel that the differential diagnosis is between pulmonary fibrosis and bronchiectasis due to the main clinical finding of bibasal crepitations on auscultation. I would try to differentiate between the two using spirometry which would demonstrate a restrictive ventilatory defect in pulmonary fibrosis but an obstructive airflow limitation in bronchiectasis. I would also request imaging in the form of chest x-ray and CT chest which may or may not reveal tram track lines and the signet ring sign in bronchiectasis or honeycombing and ground glass changes in pulmonary fibrosis.

Notice that instead of simply saying the key words of pulmonary fibrosis, bronchiectasis, spirometry, CT scan and chest x-ray, the second candidate has extended their answer to include a demonstration of their thought process and ultimately their knowledge. In exam conditions, you can never be sure what might happen – remember that both you and the examiner are under exam conditions. The examiner may or may not forget to ask a specific question in a station until time has completely ran out and you've left. Bear in mind that the examiner is also under stressful timed conditions. If they forget to ask a question and you've only answered like the first candidate, you will drop marks.

The good news is that this can be avoided by extending your answer and ensuring it's of high quality. You'll run the clock down with a longer answer hopefully dodging potentially more difficult or awkward questions that might deduct marks. I recently examined medical students during their end of year clinical OSCEs and will readily admit that I exhausted the basic questions provided by the University to ask one particularly excellent student. To avoid the awkward silence, I proceeded to ask a more nuanced question which would not be expected of her at that early stage.

More importantly you can actually steer the conversation in your preferred direction towards the knowledge you have revised. In the above example, you could easily continue the answer by talking about management of bronchiectasis and pulmonary fibrosis. Most examiners will be grateful (I was never stopped once) if you're producing a high quality and relevant answer and you're not simply rambling. I would even advocate extending each of your answers to 60 – 90 seconds long and never stopping during this time unless the examiners are visibly trying to get a word in.

"Practice makes perfect"

The second aspect of the PACES triangle is **practice**. You might be a good physician with a fountain of knowledge but the reality is that if you're unable to demonstrate this knowledge to the examiners, you'll perform poorly in MRCP PACES.

The first reason why lack of practice might fail you is when **you're unable to complete the examination stations in 6 minutes**. This is actually plenty of time to complete any one of the four major examinations and should still allow you some time to gather your thoughts before presentation and question time. However, most doctors don't carry out full respiratory examinations on each patient on their ward round and a significant number will be rusty when it comes to doing one. Even if you complete the physical examination in 5 mins 30 secs I'd recommend double checking to ensure you haven't missed any pertinent aspects, or even to assimilate your thoughts.

Secondly with practice we become **slick**. Whilst examining 1st year medical students for their end-of-year OSCEs and during our examiner training, the clinical skills tutor warned us not to automatically pass students on all modalities just because they're excellent at one or two. It's common knowledge that good-looking people are automatically assumed to be smarter, kinder and richer than those who aren't, even without good evidence. Similarly, if you're able to demonstrate slickness, examiners will automatically assume (fairly or otherwise) that you know what you're doing and that you're a great doctor even before you open your mouth to answer questions. I'm sure those assumptions are true but I can't stress enough how many extra subconscious points you'll score with the examiners if you can demonstrate a gastrointestinal examination with ease because **first impressions matter**.

So how should you structure your practice?

When practising for MRCP PACES, it's imperative to remember that although recognising pathology is important, it's absolutely necessary to nail the **normal examination** first. Understandably it's slightly awkward performing five or six of the same examination on your PACES study partner or a helpful colleague but if you have a girl/boyfriend then this shouldn't be a problem.

For the first couple of attempts, go through each and every step slowly to ensure you're ticking all the boxes. Next you can repeat this slightly quicker under timed conditions. I would encourage you to do at least ten normal examinations on each of physical examination stations 1 and 3 during the week you're studying that station. **Spread your "normal examination practice" throughout the eight weeks**. As you become more proficient and PACES draws closer, one or two examinations per week just to refresh your memory should suffice. Remember that each examination should only take 5 mins give or take.

"Presentation, presentation, presentation"

If we think back to our driving tests, even though you can drive you still have to demonstrate you're actively looking in the mirrors or checking them prior to taking off/manoeuvring. Similarly, we could theoretically navigate through the examination stations without properly understanding the significance of an ejection systolic murmur. **Presentation** is how you can demonstrate to the examiner that not only can you perform the movements, you also have the knowledge.

After passing both my written exams within the space of 3 months, my educational supervisor congratulated me. He was a very supportive consultant and gave me great advice that I write about in my first MRCP book. However, I remember one day he appeared particularly grumpy and casually mentioned out of nowhere that *"I think you might find PACES a bit difficult Rory"*. A similar thing happened with a fellow colleague. Despite being unable to clear Part 1, this colleague also directly said to me that I would struggle with PACES as it would be different from the written exams where only "hard work and study is required".

I understood why they made these comments. I'm quiet by nature as most of the time I just don't have anything to say but people can mistake this for aloofness or lack of knowledge. Fortunately, I ended up passing MRCP PACES first time using the techniques I outline in this guide. My educational supervisor was very happy for me and proudly broadcasted it to the whole hospital, but my colleague wasn't very enthusiastic!

As I have proven, leaning towards being introverted or extroverted does not determine whether you'll pass MRCP PACES or not. If you're an extrovert, I think it possibly increases your chances of passing but only if you don't ramble and go off in a tangent. If you're an introvert and you let this take over during your exam then you might be hurting your chances a little but understand that for those 2 hours and 5 minutes, you need to become a **temporary extrovert**. As I described above, even if you're an introvert, you need to extend your answer as infinitely possible to demonstrate your knowledge and determination, and also take the pressure off the examiner to ask you the next undoubtedly harder question.

How did I pass MRCP PACES with relative ease? And how did I perform so well at the ST3 interview station?

The secret really is just practice. A simple comparison would be having you sing a karaoke song tonight after a couple of ciders versus releasing a hit single. With the karaoke song you hardly have a moment's notice and the music is too loud so your voice will be drowned out. For most of us it would end in a disaster-piece. On the other hand, if you were releasing a hit single you would have hours and hours of preparation, the ability to fine tune specific portions of the song, plenty of rest and plenty of practice. The same person singing the same song, but it becomes a masterpiece.

Like most people I'm not someone who can just turn up at an event with no preparation and give a great speech or presentation. An easy way to find out whether you're gifted in this area is to imagine you've just examined a patient's cardiovascular system and you've found an irregularly irregular pulse and also a pansystolic murmur. Everything else was normal. Present to yourself in front of a mirror how you would present to an examiner under timed conditions.

If you're at the beginning of your revision you might not have given it much thought and just deliver the positive findings amongst some random negative findings. **Realise that even though you may present to your consultant or registrar every day on the ward rounds, the exam is entirely different and much more formal.**

Introverts may start off with "Mr X is a middle-aged man with an irregularly irregular pulse. On auscultation there was a pansystolic murmur. This is possibly in keeping with atrial fibrillation and mitral regurgitation" before running out of things to say. Extroverts might end up rambling but not scoring points. You want to be in that **sweet spot** where everything you say adds value to your score sheet and you want to maintain this for as long as possible.

The second point I want to touch upon was the topic of **colloquialisms** or **abbreviations**. After a few medical rotations as a FY2, CT1 and CT2, atrial fibrillation with a rapid ventricular response quickly gets shortened to *"fast AF"*. An upper gastrointestinal bleed secondary to decompensated alcoholic liver disease and portal hypertension quickly becomes abbreviated to *"upper GI bleed due to ALD"*.

In the acute medical unit this is useful because it saves us time, everyone understands each other, and also demonstrates subconsciously to the listener on the phone that you're so experienced with dealing with this condition that you can call it fast AF or ALD etc. We would never dream of calling Langerhan's Cell Histiocytosis *"LCH"* even though some respiratory specialists do!

Colloquialisms are generally frowned upon in MRCP PACES so ensure that it's chronic obstructive pulmonary disease (not COPD) and myocardial infarction (not MI). Where possible, try and be as specific as you can and this goes back to the point of **extending everything**. This means clearly stating that it's a non-ST elevation myocardial infarction. This is quite an important point and will need some time getting used to. When was the last time you said to your colleague even something as straightforward as "atrial fibrillation" in full?

To shift your mindset in the lead up towards the exam, begin writing the full version of every condition in your clerk-ins in the acute medical unit. In the superficial exam setting, you will make yourself sound much more eloquent. Fast AF sounds very silly if you think about it and could actually mean fast as f***!

The last point I wanted to mention about presentation is to actually practice presenting. I would highly encourage you to invest in a **dictaphone** or a **voice recording application** on your smartphone. If you hate the sound of your own voice being played back, then you're not alone. I think most of us do but there's no other solution to overcoming this.

For the above example of the irregularly irregular pulse and pansystolic murmur, start your preparation by imagining how you would present whilst you're on your commute or if you have a few minutes at work. Ideally you could present to a PACES partner but if it's your first attempt even that can be quite intimidating. When you're alone, present the case fully and as clearly as possible to the voice recorder and **replay it back to yourself**. **Critique yourself** and truly listen for stuttering or pertinent pieces of information being missed.

When you start off you may sound like this:

"I have just examined Mr X who is a...seventy um...something year old gentleman. He is comfortable at rest and is not in respiratory distress. On examination I found an irregularly irregular pulse at 84 beats per minute and a pansystolic murmur radiating to the axilla. This is probably mitral regurgitation associated with AF."

As you progress you'll soon sound like this:

"Mr X is an elderly gentleman who has kindly let me examine him. His main positive findings include an irregularly irregular pulse at 84 beats per minute and a pansystolic murmur radiating to the axilla. There was no clinical evidence of infective endocarditis, heart failure or anticoagulation. This is most likely mitral regurgitation associated with atrial fibrillation. Differentials of a pansystolic murmur can also include tricuspid regurgitation and ventricular septal defect and if I had time I would like to proceed to history taking and full respiratory examination. In terms of investigations, a 12 lead electrocardiogram would be useful to confirm atrial fibrillation. An echocardiogram would be important to characterise the valvular defect. If atrial fibrillation is confirmed then calculating the CHADSVASC score to stratify stroke risk would be my priority as this would guide anticoagulation therapy..."

Firstly, avoid trying to guess a patient's age. I've been in medicine for almost ten years now and I still frequently get it wrong. If the patient is young, call them young. If they're old, call them elderly. And if they're in between, call them middle aged. **Always be generous** though because you don't want to insult the examiner!

Secondly, every station has **important negatives**. In the above cardiology station, it is important to mention the lack of clinical evidence of anticoagulation such as ecchymoses as you would expect patients with known AF to be on anticoagulation.

Thirdly, always present your most likely diagnosis first. PACES cases are usually imperfect as it's not easy identifying "standard patients". In cases of mixed valvular disease, even the examiners have to rely on the echocardiogram report.

This is the reason why we follow up our most likely diagnosis with a differential. You should also continue (without pause) on **how you would differentiate between your differential diagnosis** because that is clearly the next question. If you were the examiner and the candidate gave three possible answers, you'd want them to narrow down the differential. Essentially, we are trying to predict their questions and make the process as easy as possible. I never did this for my preparation but you might want to consider writing down a candidate versus examiner interaction to hopefully place you in the shoes of the examiner. This may help you predict the next question.

Invest in a great course

"No-one fails after going to this course Rory"

Up until now I had never attended a course for any exam but MRCP PACES was admittedly a little different to any exam I had been to before. Everyone was raving about this London PACES course. I don't advertise other people's products (nor am I getting paid to do so) but in the interests of providing you with the best information I know about this topic, the course I attended was **PassPACES**. From memory I think the course organiser at the time was Rupa Bessant a rheumatologist.

The exam costs about £700 but this course was double. *Do I really need it?* The price of the four-day course was a whopping £1,395 and in London that's the least of your worries. Accommodation, travel and subsistence brought that figure well over £2,000- or essentially more than one-month's salary as a CT1. As I write this in June 2020 the course alone now costs £1,495.

I deliberated some more before deciding I couldn't afford it and applied for the local hospital's PACES course instead. After all, it would cost one month's salary and I still had rent and food to pay for. A few weeks before the local PACES course was due to start, it was cancelled due to insufficient delegate numbers and I immediately seized the opportunity to request for the trust to pay for this London PACES course. Although I still ended up paying over £500 for accommodation and food, I'm very grateful my trust paid for this course. The lesson from this story is *if you don't ask you don't get*. We should always request study leave allowance first before paying for courses ourselves because each trust receives money from their national education department to invest in us.

If your hospital hosts their own PACES course then it'll be difficult to justify them spending so much money but keep your eyes peeled for any opportunities that may arise.

The fully booked four-day course was very intense and spanned most of each day between 8am and 5pm. There were countless patients with a wide range of pathology available for getting practical experience on. I actually took quite unwell after day 1 but because so much money was involved, I powered on for the remaining three days.

The organiser was very strict and the environment was so stressful that one of the candidates disappeared after day 2. For the days he was present he was very nervous and struggled during presentations. Personally I loved every minute of it because I felt like I was training for something really important, almost like in some type of boot camp. In reality, it's quite hard to justify spending £2,000 on top of the PACES fee but there is a reason why this course is always fully booked.

Over the four days I saw a multitude of pathology and in fact one of the cases (**simultaneous pancreatic and kidney transplant**) actually appeared in the exam. Having never done a renal SHO job before, I had never encountered this presentation until then so I'm really glad I attended the course.

You don't have to attend that specific course obviously but I've still yet to come across someone who bravely skips a PACES course before their exam. There are shorter two-day courses available for half the price so that's an alternative option but I'll let you do your own research on this one.

Weeks 1 and 2

Hopefully by now you have a good overview of what it takes to pass MRCP PACES. In addition to having a solid knowledge base, you'll need to demonstrate sound organisational skills by structuring your preparation in 8 weeks around your busy CMT jobs.

We discussed the need to revise using a good PACES book to gain PACES-specific knowledge rapidly. We stressed the importance of practising examination skills and ultimately presentation skills with aid of a voice recording tool.

Now we must think about the structure of your revision in the upcoming eight weeks.

In **week 1**, I would advise working on **respiratory and abdominal** examination using the PACES triangle. In **week 2** you might then focus on the **cardiology and neurology** stations. Your first week might look something like this:

> Mon – Respiratory
> Tues – Abdominal
> Wed – Respiratory
> Thurs – Abdominal
> Fri – Respiratory
> Sat – Abdominal
> Sun – Resp & Abdo

Following from above, your respiratory revision might then look like this:

Mon
Read PACES-specific knowledge book for 2 hours; Practice respiratory examination for 30 minutes; practice presenting a respiratory condition for 30 minutes e.g. lobectomy & pleural effusion

Wed
Read PACES-specific knowledge book for 2 hours; Practice respiratory examination for 10 minutes; practice presenting a respiratory condition for 30 minutes e.g. COPD & bronchiectasis

Fri
Read PACES-specific knowledge book for 2 hours; Practice respiratory examination for 5 minutes; practice presenting a respiratory condition for 30 minutes e.g. TB

Sun
Read PACES-specific knowledge book for 1 hour; Practice respiratory examination for 5 minutes; practice presenting a respiratory condition for 15 minutes e.g. transplant

Regardless of whether you have 2, 8 or 16 weeks before MRCP PACES it's always a good idea to set your revision timetable roughly like this before you dive in just to ensure you cover the required material in equal amounts. If you were to follow the above plan for example, you would've carried out 7 hours of knowledge studying, just under 2 hours of presentation practice and just under an hour of physical examination practice for a total of 10 hours. This would be for the typical internal medicine trainee who is working 48 hours a week and should be adjusted if you are on night shift etc. Most trainees would have nowhere near 2 hours of presentation practice per specialty and it will show during the exam.

Here, it is important to recall the concept of **study variation**. Reading for 2 hours from a textbook can become dull very quickly so your Monday might consist of reading for 1 hour, practising for 20 minutes, presenting for 20 minutes, reading for 1 hour, practising for 10 minutes and presenting for 10 minutes. Remember at some point during this (preferably the earlier the better) you should start presenting to your colleagues (and not just to yourself or the voice recorder). Likewise, you should start examining real patients to attempt to differentiate between different murmurs etc.

Remember not to excuse yourself from practising a full respiratory examination just because you're not in the hospital or there happens to be no patients with that physical sign on that day. A normal respiratory examination under timed conditions is sometimes just as good. With some stretch of imagination, you can "pretend" your PACES partner has a lobectomy scar or right sided crackles and just present these made-up findings for presentation practice. That's essentially what you'll find in a pneumonectomy or lobectomy. Being able to perform the examination with slickness and within 6 minutes is so much more important.

While 10 hours might seem like a lot of hours, anxious candidates may look at this study plan and feel that it's careless or even slightly short. I highly respect people who are grafters which is why I try to stay on the treadmill for an hour each time, but I am so quite realistic. Even during a normal working day, you only have between 7 – 11pm to study. Factor in on calls including night shifts and the 20 hours a week of studying (remember resp and abdo) becomes very arduous if not impossible. The sensible amongst you might choose to sit MRCP PACES during a less intense block, during a less intense period of their rota or even taking annual leave. Parkinson's Law is also always in action meaning that if you have a set amount of time e.g. 8 weeks to pass MRCP PACES then you'll use 8 weeks. If you're given one year then you'll use the full year – in reality, you'll never be "ready" so it's better to grit your teeth and carry on ahead.

Begin your revision by spending 40 hours over 14 days studying respiratory, abdominal, cardiology and neurology and ensure that you move onto the next phase of revision even if you don't feel 100% ready. You'll have time at the end of the eight weeks to revisit areas that you feel are lacking.

The table below highlights the main aspects you'll be tested on in the physical examination stations.

Physical examination stations
Comprehensive and correct physical examination technique
Detect physical signs
Construct differential diagnosis
Suggest sensible and appropriate investigation and management plans
Treat patient with dignity and respect

Week 3

"Medicine is 90% history and 10% examination"

In real life clinical practice, the majority of the diagnosis comes from history and investigations. Physical examination rarely clinches a diagnosis unless it's an obvious rash like psoriasis or an acute abdomen for example. Following on from Parts I and II however, MRCP PACES does not mimic real life!

Your third week should be spent honing history taking and communication skills. The acute medical take is quite often filled with issues related to frailty, respiratory exacerbations and decompensated cardiac and endocrine diseases. Whilst you'll already be slick with history taking patients who attend with the bread-and-butter conditions, you might find some aspects of history taking awkward, or find ethical scenarios tricky. Be sure to know and use the up-to-date terms such as "PWID" which stands for "person who injects drugs" rather than the outdated "IVDU", "MSM" which stands for "man who has sex with other men" rather than "homosexual". Also, ensure you're comfortable with taking a sexual history or asking about the menstrual cycle.

Remember that it is not enough to *think* you can take a sexual history – the words that come out of your mouth during the start of your practice may surprise you. A useful technique is simply to be honest and upfront before asking your awkward question. "Apologies for asking this question which might seem strange, but you'll see that it's very relevant to your symptoms."

In addition to being able to manoeuvre your way around awkwardness slickly you'll also be required to identify so-called **key differentiating questions**. An example of a key differentiating question would be asking about a patient's occupation when they present with obstructive sleep apnoea. In the current history taking station 2 you should aim to pick up most marks because although in real life clinical practice you may only spend 30 seconds listening to someone's chest on the ward round, it's not entirely unusual to speak to someone for 30 minutes. By sheer relative time spent on history taking versus examination, this should be a strength and therefore all that you need to do is to hone your skills.

Your week 3 might look something like this:

Mon – Respiratory
Tues – Dermatology/Opthalmology/Psychiatry
Wed – Geriatrics/Neurology
Thurs – Cardiology
Fri – Haematology/Oncology/Palliative
Sat – Gastroenterology/Renal
Sun – GUM/infectious diseases/drugs

For each major condition in each specialty, you might wish to think about some key differentiating questions and any ethical situations you might face. For example, obstructive sleep apnoea in a long-distance HGV driver is a classical one. Another would be the issue of compensation in asbestosis/mesothelioma. The knowledge PACES book that I recommended earlier should cover some of this, but any good textbook or online resource will help.

The main point is to differentiate yourself from a medical student taking a history. Anyone can take a good chest pain history using the SOCRATES acronym but in PACES they're testing whether you can create a reasonable differential diagnosis following your history. They also want to know whether you're able to stratify this chest pain into low, medium or high risk. What implications does this have? Does the patient need admitting or can they have outpatient investigations? Whilst SOCRATES is useful in a headache history, you'll also want to know if there are any features of increased intracranial pressure. Every history taking station has its own set of differentiating questions so remember it's not simply a tick box exercise of asking about their family history, smoking, alcohol and social history.

The best strategy is to ask questions slowly but also simultaneously ask yourself what condition this could be. What are the differentials? What is the key issue(s) the examiners are wanting me to address?

Throughout week 3 you should also practice each of the four major clinical examinations: respiratory, neurology, cardiology and abdominal once just to maintain your slickness. That should only take you 20 mins for all four but well worth the time.

History taking
Gather data from patient
Construct a differential diagnosis
Deal with concerns the patient may have
Construct a management plan that is explained to the patient clearly
Treat patient with dignity and respect

The above table documents the main areas examiners are assessing you in during history taking.

There are 16 sample history taking stations on the MRCP(UK) website which you might find useful.

Creating systematic presentations

Knowledge, Practice and Presentation are your three main pillars for MRCP PACES success.

By now hopefully you've either invested in a voice recording device or downloaded an equivalent application on your phone. You'll have had time to practice in front of the mirror and unless you're naturally good at presenting patients in a systematic manner, hopefully you'll realise there's a lot of work to be done!

The reason why you want to create systematic presentations at this point in your revision is because now you have an overall idea of what the exam is about. You have also had a chance to revise history taking and physical examination for the major four systems and hopefully have had a look at some of the minor ones.

It cannot be stressed enough that it's worth spending an hour or so drafting up a systematic presentation for each organ system. For example, when presenting in a **renal** station, you want to ask yourself a pre-determined set of questions and this goes for all the history taking and physical examination stations. Here's an example of how your thought process might look like:

1. What is the aetiology? The main causes of renal failure are hypertension and diabetes, but you'll need to remember vasculitis, polycystic kidney disease and a couple of rare ones. When examining, state you would like to check the BP and perform a finger prick test or

simply look for them on the patient's fingers! When history taking, do not just ask for a general family history, ask specifically for autosomal dominant polycystic kidney disease!
2. Current renal replacement therapy (RRT)?
3. Previous RRT? The common forms of RRT are renal transplant, haemodialysis (via fistulae or central venous catheter) and peritoneal dialysis. Therefore, always look for scars in the abdomen, neck and the anterior chest. Gently palpate for a mass under the scar.
4. Is the RRT working or not? Only stable patients are used for PACES examinations and therefore 99/100 times you'll only need to mention that the RRT is working. Often times it may feel like stating the obvious but like in a driving test, you have to make your thought process evident to the examiner.
5. Any complications? This is where it can get slightly confusing. Essentially you want to think about what medications a patient on RRT would be taking. Corticosteroids, ciclosporin and tacrolimus are the most common ones but be aware of others. Not only can finger prick marks alert you to the aetiology of end stage renal failure, bear in mind that some immunosuppressants can lead to diabetes. This is an area where you can potentially impress the examiners.

The reason why I've specifically mentioned the renal station is because although we've performed the neurology or abdominal examinations since early medical school, I don't recall being specifically taught a renal examination.

Bringing all this together, your presentation might sound like this (and it's worth reciting this out loud a few times): "Mr X is a middle-aged gentleman presenting with... This gentleman most likely has end stage renal failure with a renal transplant. The aetiology is most likely diabetes mellitus due to the presence of fingertip prick marks indicative of blood glucose monitoring, but differential diagnoses would include hypertension and vasculitis. His current renal replacement therapy is a functioning right renal transplant as evidenced by a right iliac fossa scar with an underlying smooth and firm mass dull to percussion. The presence of a non-functioning brachiocephalic fistula in his left arm suggests previous haemodialysis. There are no other scars on the anterior chest wall, neck or abdomen to suggest other forms of renal replacement therapy. The renal transplant appears to be functioning well due to Mr X's euvolaemic state and absence of confusion and asterixis. The presence of gum hypertrophy may also suggest that this gentleman is taking an immunosuppressant such as ciclosporin. To complete my assessment I would like to take a full history and perform bedside investigations such as a urinalysis to look for microscopic haematuria, proteinuria and glucose. I would also like to check his haematological and biochemical profile with FBC, U&Es, CK, HCO_3, HbA1c....and imaging in the form of renal tract ultrasound..."

There are a multitude of ways to continue with this presentation and you might wish to experiment. For example, why not practise presenting an imaginary patient who is being haemodialysed via peritoneal dialysis? You can continue the presentation by explaining what you're looking for with blood tests and ultrasound. Try not to let your presentation stop unless you've exhausted your bank of useful information or you notice your examiners trying to ask you a new question.

Remember end stage renal failure is not a diagnosis – you'll be expected to come up with a cause!

Weeks 4, 5 and 6

In weeks 4, 5 and 6 you should start preparing holistically for the brief clinical encounters station 5 which will comprise a third of the entire exam's marks. These are the stations that most mimic real-life clinical practice. For instance, if you have 8 weeks to study for PACES you should dedicate around 3 weeks to these stations alone.

The best resources I'd recommend are the above **PACES course, videos** and the textbook **An Aid to the MRCP PACES by Ryder Station 5 Volume 3**.

Station 5 consist of two 10-minute clinical encounters attempting to simulate to the examiners how you would interact with a patient in real life. The good news is that you should already be familiar with this type of format in real life clinical practice – all you have left to do is to hone your skills and slickness by "combining" history taking/communication and physical examination into one. Due to time restraints, every question and examination section should be focussed.

The other difficulty with station 5 rests upon how to practice and present cases. After reading about the PACES triangle you might have a better appreciation of the work required to properly structure your presentation and answer when it comes to **major medical systems** such as respiratory and neurology. There's a clear linear thought process that you can demonstrate to the examiner to confirm your knowledge, practice and presentation skills. How can we do that in a focussed way in station 5?

This is where I think the Ryder textbook is a lifesaver, and the following was how I used that book.

The book begins with an examination routine section where it teaches you a systematic way of examining seemingly random but very relevant **minor systems** such as pulses, fundi, hands and even skin. Most internal medicine trainees probably haven't had many opportunities to attend dermatology or ophthalmology clinics, and how many of those that have done so actually learned to present one of these minor systems formally? Having a systematic routine to examine the skin or the eyes is invaluable – the bottom line is that even if you're unable to identify the rash or see anything during fundoscopy, being able to describe you process will demonstrate to the examiners you understand what you're doing.

After you learn the formal way of examining each minor system, the PACES triangle states you should now practice doing this. For example, practice the thyroid examination enough times so that reaching for that tendon hammer is second nature. Again, this does not necessitate finding a patient with a goitre – you can practice all the moves on a PACES partner prior to finding a real patient. This means performing this examination several occasions initially on your partner and maintaining this slickness throughout your eight weeks.

And once you're comfortable with performing the examination, you should now start working on presentation.

A resource is only as good as the student, just like a tool or weapon is only as good as the person wielding it. I suspect most candidates read the Ryder textbook passively and find the examinations and presentations of dermatomyositis, for example, interesting. But if the candidate doesn't practice the "dermatomyositis examination" and has never presented such a case before, how can they expect to come across as capable in the exam? Remember that it is worthwhile presenting a few hypothyroidism or dermatomyositis presentations to your voice recorder app and partner.

Always remember that PACES revision should be **30% input and 70% output**. 30% of the time can be spent on **consumption** activities such as reading textbooks and watching videos – these are passive actions that most candidates are adept at doing. The remaining **productive** 70% of your time should be used effectively to produce movement and voice; movement in the form of practising the examination skills you learn from textbooks/videos and voice in the form of honing your presentation skills.

Initially you may open the book and be overwhelmed by the sheer number of cases, but one piece of good news is that you only need to learn one examination routine for each minor system. Regardless of whether the patient has retinitis pigmentosa or diabetic retinopathy, your ophthalmology examination framework will always be the same.

On the topic of examination practice, it's important not to make excuses or create imaginary barriers. For example, if you don't have access to an ophthalmoscope that evening, consider using a pen and practice all the other movements on your partner, making sure you use your right eye to examine their right eye and so on. Even becoming slicker with your instructions to the patient such as always asking them to look "up, left, right then down" will come across during the PACES exam, and the only way to do this is to practice. The ophthalmoscopy findings only play a portion of the station so not having access should not preclude you from beginning your practice. When you do have access to an ophthalmoscope, you can now concentrate on how to adjust its settings and switch it on etc.

Finally, in relation to the Ryder book, after reading the initial patient clinical encounter paragraph, I would advise covering the author's presentation and answers. Reading the examination findings once and then presenting the case out loud followed by reading the author's standard presentation afterwards and compare their written response to your verbal one is a useful exercise. Do this enough and certain key phrases become second nature. Not only do you now have the knowledge, you can also demonstrate this through rehearsed presentation skills.

In addition to a PACES course and Ryder's book, I would also recommend using a PACES website to give your revision some variety. Active effort such as presentation and practising will always be more difficult to the passive learning of material i.e. reading books and watching videos. The former is also difficult because you're opening yourself to another person's judgement. However, through active effort is where you truly improve as the PACES candidate.

As such I would always start my revision each day with active activities such as those in the PACES triangle. When you're exhausted from reading, practising and presenting, you have the option to watch one of your predecessors perform the examination under standard and timed conditions. From my experience, the website with the best videos is **Pastest**. One advantage of watching other people is that you can incorporate their good habits into your routine whilst ensuring you oust their bad ones.

There are 9 station 5 sample scenarios on the MRCP(UK) website which you might find useful.

Weeks 7 and 8

The timetable for your final two weeks will be very dependent on how your revision has gone so far. For each of the first six weeks, regardless of whether you're ready or not, I would strongly urge you to continue to the next stage of revision as the likelihood is that you'll never feel ready because medicine is just such a vast topic. Even still hopefully you've managed to cover all of the major and most of the minor stations by now. The last two weeks will be to clean up anything you feel you've missed or are worried about.

Note that a common condition in PACES does not necessarily mean common in real life. An example of this would be acromegaly which comes up relatively frequently in the exam but hardly ever in hospital. Your response to this should be to read, practice and present a few acromegaly cases!

I would spend a few days during weeks 7 and 8 on communication skills. For most current practising doctors, this should be relatively straightforward. During my station 4 I was counselling a woman on her father who was slowly dying from the complications associated with Parkinson's disease. Although it requires you to have some knowledge of the condition so that you steer the consultation in the right direction, most of the scenario revolves around your ability to elicit the daughter's **ideas, concerns and expectations (ICE)** so even a lay person can score highly in those areas.

Communication station
Guide and organise the interview with the subject
Explain clinical information
Apply clinical knowledge, including ethics, to management of case or situation
Provide emotional support
Treat the patient with dignity and respect

It should go without saying that communication skills are much more than this so you'll need to brush up on your structure of **how to deliver bad news** and reinforce your knowledge on basic concepts like the **mental health act, confidentiality and the four bioethical principles** for example. There are 24 communication skills and ethics sample scenarios on the MRCP(UK) website which you might find useful.

Otherwise your last two weeks should be spent plugging any perceived holes you may have in your knowledge, practice and presentation of the major and minor systems. If you're not too confident in differentiating between an ejection systolic and pansystolic murmur, now is the time to seek the help of a friendly cardiologist. If all rashes look the same, then now's the time to revisit that chapter of the Ryder book. The next day you could visit the dermatology ward or clinic for some practice.

Most importantly, be honest and critical of yourself. If your pauses are too long during presentation, spend the next week presenting one hundred cases!

MRCP PACES Marking Scheme

At the beginning of the exam you'll be given 16 marksheets with verbal instructions to write your name and candidate number on each. Although there are only 5 stations, there are 8 separate scenarios (see table) and two examiners at each scenario, totalling 16 (some will be duplicates). Learning the marking scheme is learning to play the game so to speak.

Station	Scenario	Examiners
1	Respiratory Abdominal	A + B
2	History taking	C + D
3	Neurology Cardiology	E + F
4	Communication skills	G + H
5	Brief Clinical Encounter 1 Brief Clinical Encounter 2	I + J

7 separate skills are assessed in MRCP PACES and each scenario tests a different combination of these skills. In reality, the marks are essentially binary and can be summarised as follows.

If you're deemed unsatisfactory in a particular skill, the examiner will designate you 0 marks; borderline and you're given a 1 and if you're satisfactory then you're awarded 2 marks. It is important to note that you only have to be satisfactory, and that there are no extra points for being excellent.

The second table details the seven skills that you'll be assessed on and the minimum pass marks required:

	Skills	Pass mark
A	Physical examination	16/24
B	Identifying physical signs	14/24
C	Clinical communication	11/16
D	Differential diagnosis	17/28
E	Clinical Judgement	19/32
F	Managing patient concerns	10/16
G	Maintaining patient welfare	28/32
	Total pass mark required	130/172

So, to attain MRCP PACES, you'll need to score 130 out of the available 172 marks <u>and</u> pass each separate skill individually. For example, if a candidate scored 138/172 but only managed 13/24 in skill B then this would unfortunately still equate to a fail. The other caveat is that a candidate who scores 28/32 in skill G – the examiners will assess your overall performance and decide whether you pass or not, regardless of your total test score. This is because maintaining patient welfare are basic requirements of being a courteous professional. These will include ensuring the patient is not in pain during your physical examination, and you show empathy during a difficult communication for instance. Here are the individual skills in more detail:

	Clinical skill	Descriptor
A	Examination	Correct, thorough, systematic, fluent and professional technique
B	Identifying signs	Correctly. Do not find signs that aren't there
C	Communication	Elicit relevant, systematic, thorough, fluent and professional history. Explain

			information similarly
D		Differential diagnosis	Sensible
E		Judgement	Select or negotiate sensible management plan. Select appropriate investigations or treatments. Apply clinical knowledge and ethics.
F		Managing concerns	Seek, detect, acknowledge and address concerns. Listen and demonstrate empathy
G		Maintaining welfare	Respect, comfort, safety and dignity

It is worth spending some time looking at the individual words of the above table and contemplating how you'll demonstrate to the examiner each of these. The examiner will have a similar marking sheet in front of them and although they'll be encouraged to write notes for feedback, the most important part is the binary tick box.

Under skill A, it is important you follow the PACES triangle and practise the correct technique enough times so that you can demonstrate this to the examiner in a thorough and systematic manner whilst maintaining slickness (fluency). For skill G, perhaps it is worthwhile spending 10 seconds to greet the patient and ask what their preferred (nick)name is. Everyone appreciates that you're a respectful person but how can you show this to the examiner? Do this for each skill and you will get a better understanding of how to approach the exam.

Station	Encounter	Skills assessed
1	Respiratory Abdomen	A B D E G

2	History taking	C D E F G
3	Cardiovascular Neurology	A B D E G
4	Communication	C E F G
5	Brief clinical encounter (1) Brief clinical encounter (2)	A B C D E F G

This next table is also worth a look. Station 5 assesses you on all 7 skills; each skill is worth 2 marks and there are two examiners and two stations. Therefore, a total of 56/172 marks will come from this station alone. This is the reason why we dedicate 3/8 weeks of our study plan to the brief clinical encounters.

As mentioned, not only is excelling in skill G paramount to your success in MRCP PACES, it is also a skill that is present throughout all 5 stations. They comprise 32/172 marks so ensure you don't drop any easy marks! Interestingly, skill E is also present in all the stations which is why I would advise creating a solid presentation framework and taking the initiative to demonstrate to the examiner your management plan, investigations and treatment options, instead of passively waiting for the examiner to ask you each question in turn.

Apart from the challenging station 5, the other main stumbling block is the so-called **linked** skills, namely B, D and E. For instance, if a candidate incorrectly identifies a cardiac murmur that isn't present, they'll marked down on their ability to identify physical signs. Their presumption of an imaginary murmur might then mislead them to incorrectly list aortic stenosis as one of their differentials, and the erroneous investigation of choice to be an echocardiogram. You can see why identifying the wrong physical sign caused this candidate to lose marks (potentially 12) in skills B, D and E so it is worth spending some time on.

Read the scenario. Then read it again.

In addition to having been through the journey myself not too long ago (2015), I have been the organising registrar for two formal MRCP PACES exams. I have also participated as an examiner in one the MRCP PACES courses in Hull.

The main thing that struck me in all the encounters was the number of candidates who failed to read the question properly. Unfortunately, it demonstrates to the examiner a lackadaisical attitude even if the candidate is struggling to read the question fully with limited time. Quite often it is worth asking the examiner for an extra 30 seconds to read over the scenario before you formally start your station but beware that the clock is ticking! Many scenarios are lengthy, but you can usually take the question sheet into the station and refer to it anytime. No marks will be deducted for apologising to the patient and referring to the question sheet that might contain useful clinical details like BP, cholesterol level and how many cats and dogs the patient has.

Clinical vignettes that have multiple bullet points or stems are used to prompt candidates. For example, a communication station such as the end-stage Parkinson's disease one may ask you to:

- Explain the situation to the daughter
- Propose any treatments
- Advise on prognosis

You'll need to prioritise these three aspects of the consultation to maximise your marks but also bearing in mind the marking scheme that we discussed. Failing to address one of them is akin to automatically surrendering a third of your marks for that station.

Non-technical skills

It's worth paying some attention to the non-technical skills that can increase your chances of success by 5 – 10% on a given day. A significant proportion of candidates revise consistently for months on end whilst holding busy banded jobs, but this can be a recipe for burnout. I firmly believe in resting your mind and letting yourself recover during these much-needed rest periods.

It goes without saying that nutrition, exercise and sleep all play an important role in how you will perform on the day. Ensure you're drinking plenty of water, doing some form of cardiovascular exercise and sleeping plenty in the lead up to the exam. Anything else that can be optimised beforehand should be – prior to becoming a medical registrar it is worthwhile investing in a better stethoscope. Even if it might not increase your chances of hearing a cardiac murmur by 2% (it might), it'll surely help you in your future career. A new and comfortable shirt or dress might also be indicated for the same reasons for those who need an excuse to spend money...

It can also be useful to research your PACES centre to see what their "specialty" is, because most hospitals are famous for being good at something. Even if you only live 30 minutes away from the hospital, it's worth paying for a hotel and staying close by your PACES centre the night before. Don't underestimate the effect of being stuck in traffic for one hour will have on your feelings and performance. Try and ensure everything is accounted for including your dinner the night before, the breakfast before the exam and your parking space etc. Will there be taxis on Monday at 830am?

PACES Fast Track & Failing

If you've applied for ST3 then it is worth applying for PACES fast track simultaneously when you apply for MRCP PACES. Although spaces are very limited, it is worth having two bites at the cherry as there are many factors that can influence success or failure. If you pass the original sitting, then they will refund your money on the fast track exam but failing the original gives you a second opportunity to pass and obtain your MRCP diploma and ST3 post.

It is always advisable to resit immediately if you feel you were well prepared but some factor outside your control negatively influenced your result. I cannot stress the importance of requesting **detailed feedback** from the examiners. Whilst you're waiting for their reply, take a few days off everything to **reflect** on anything you could've improved upon. Without being hyper self-critical, if you're terrible at recognising rashes then spend a disproportionately large amount of your clinic time in the dermatology department prior to your next sitting. If English isn't your first language and you think that played a major part in your hamartia then from now until your next exam, speak nothing but English even if it's outside your comfort zone.

If you have any questions or comments, please don't hesitate to contact me via **rory@ukdoctoronfire.com**. I look forward to hearing from you. Good luck!

Printed in Great Britain
by Amazon